Statutory and Mandatory Training in Health and Social Care

Wendy Garcarz
Managing Director
4 Health Ltd

and

Emma Wilcock
Education and Learning Manager
Stoke-on-Trent Teaching PCT Programme

Radcliffe Publishing
Oxford • Seattle

Radcliffe Publishing Ltd
18 Marcham Road
Abingdon
Oxon OX14 1AA
United Kingdom

www.radcliffe-oxford.com
Electronic catalogue and worldwide online ordering facility.

British Library Cataloguing in Publication Data

A catalogue record for this book is available from the British Library.

ISBN 1 85775 686 X

Typeset by Aarontype Ltd, Easton, Bristol
Printed and bound by TJ International Ltd, Padstow, Cornwall

Contents

Preface

Organisations are required by law to ensure that their staff undertake training specific to the nature of their working environment (statutory training), for example health & safety training, fire lectures, etc. In addition, responsible organisations publish a list of their standard requirements for key skills training (mandatory training) which they consider essential to their workforce.

Through the work I have done with many health and social care-related organisations, I have often identified a 'laissez faire' approach to this subject. Some organisations regard this as a 'tick-box' exercise where proof of attendance or update is taken as proof of competence.

This toolkit sets out the risks involved in such an approach and establishes strong arguments for strengthening policy and practice in such organisations. The focus of the toolkit is to promote as good practice the measurement of competence in these statutory and mandatory training areas.

The checklists and templates as shown in the Appendices to this toolkit are available for readers to print off at www.radcliffe-oxford.com/statmand.

Wendy Garcarz
4 Health Ltd
January 2005

About the authors

Wendy Garcarz MA, DipEd, DipTM is Managing Director of 4 Health Ltd, a change management consultancy company working with public sector organisations to achieve sustainable change through workforce development. Wendy is an educationalist with more than 20 years' experience, specialising in organisational development and creating learning organisations. For further details visit their website: www.4-health.biz

Emma Wilcock is the Education and Learning Manager with the Stoke-on-Trent Teaching Primary Care Trust Programme. She has worked in learning and development for the last six years, having begun her career as a solicitor. Emma has experience of managing professional development requirements in a variety of regulated sectors, including health, financial services and the law. She has a particular interest in linking training to competence in practice.

Acknowledgements

The authors would like to thank:

- Sara Rogers, Training Co-ordinator, Burntwood, Lichfield and Tamworth PCT, for her significant contribution to the content of the toolkit
- Stoke on Trent Teaching PCT for their support in developing and testing the content of the toolkit.

Purpose of the toolkit

This toolkit will offer a framework for:

- establishing organisational standards for statutory and mandatory training
- identifying training needs of the workforce
- clarifying which areas of practice require statutory, mandatory training and proven competence[1] and which skills and subject areas this applies to, including:
  - core courses that carry statutory and mandatory status
  - staff groups' specific requirements for statutory and mandatory training
- developing processes for identification of need, measurement of competence and monitoring status
- quality assurance of externally and internally provided training programmes by defining quality criteria for learning activities.

The toolkit also:

- identifies a number of practical tools and templates to assist in the development and implementation of sound statutory and mandatory training practice in an organisation.

The toolkit offers guidance for:

- secondary and specialist NHS trusts wishing to review their existing policy and provision

---

[1] Department of Health (2000) *Improving Working Lives*. DoH, London.

- primary care trusts that need to promote and provide statutory and mandatory training for their workforce and support independent contractors and their employed staff
- independent contractors providing services in the health or social care sectors, i.e. dentists, general practitioners, chiropodists, pharmacists, etc.
- care organisations that provide patient/user services and that are subject to external inspection or regulation, i.e. residential/care homes, day centres, etc.
- all employees (managers and staff) to help determine the mandatory and statutory training relevant to each individual and to identify the most effective method of delivery.

Section 1:

Rationale for statutory and mandatory training

Introduction

Organisations have legal responsibilities to provide a safe and healthy environment for their staff, subcontractors and visiting members of the public. They are required to provide a range of training that ensures that their workforce has the correct level of knowledge and skill to operate safely and that a safe and healthy working environment is maintained. Although there is legislation that requires statutory training to be identified, organisations need to establish their own minimum standards for safe practice tailored to their business demands and requirements.

By publishing their mandatory training requirements, they are establishing an organisational standard that offers clarity for the workforce and ensures consistency and quality in their provision of statutory and mandatory training.

This toolkit has been developed to support organisations in reviewing their current arrangements and establishing sound statutory and mandatory training practice throughout their organisation. Through the toolkit they can develop policy, minimum standards, subsequent implementation and robust monitoring systems that place significant emphasis on competence development, not simply attendance of sessions. There are tools, exercises and checklists that can be used with individuals, teams or across the whole workforce to ensure that statutory and mandatory training is integral to individual development and quality service delivery.

The legal requirement for statutory and mandatory training

Statutory training is determined by legislation including the Health & Safety at Work Act 1974, the Employment Relations Act 1999 and the Race Relations Amendment Act 2000. Mandatory training includes skills and knowledge training for all staff (some specific to certain staff groups and disciplines) and this is determined by the organisation's policies, government guidelines and sector specifications.

Each function or profession may also contribute to determining its mandatory requirements. This information needs to be integrated into the corporate planning and education commissioning cycles and should ultimately form part of the learning needs analysis, staff appraisal and personal development plans.

Training and development activities are not restricted to traditional forms of training courses but include a variety of methods and approaches that offer staff flexible access to statutory and mandatory training.

Establishing statutory and mandatory training standards in an organisation

It is vital that organisations understand their legal requirements in order to fully comply with them. The Workplace (Health, Safety & Welfare) Regulations 1992 cover the six key areas of health & safety regulations governing a wide range of organisations: Health & Safety in the Workplace; Risk Assessment; COSHH; RIDDOR; Fire Safety; Electrical Testing.

Employers have a duty under the Health & Safety at Work Act 1974 to take reasonable measures to ensure the health, safety and welfare of their employees at work. They also have a duty towards people who are not their employees but who use their premises. The implications of failure to comply with the regulations are extremely serious and can result in premises closure or significant fines being levied against the organisation. In a serious breech of statutory regulations, responsible individuals may be personally culpable and this can result in fines or even jail terms being given if the organisation is found guilty.

The regulations aim to ensure that the health, safety and welfare requirements of the workforce are met (including those with disabilities). Regulations make it very clear that measures taken by the organisation should be suitable and applicable for anyone. As an example, this means that public access, toilets and workstations need to cater for those with special physical/learning needs.

To ensure that this happens, the organisation puts in place policies and procedures which outline the standard expected and the method of achieving that standard but that is only part of the process. The organisation then needs to ensure that all employees understand and implement the policies in a consistent way to be certain that practice mirrors policy.

There are a number of methods employed to do this:

- induction training for all new members of staff (*see* Appendix 1 for checklist)
- employee handbooks that contain the necessary information
- statutory and mandatory training stipulated by the organisation as necessary for the job/role
- team briefing as a mechanism for updating, reviewing and informing the workforce of changes to the policies.

The organisation will need to make some decisions about what it considers essential learning for its staff and establish standards covering those areas. The key questions are:

- what needs to be done to meet requirements and regulations? (statutory)
  and

- what does the organisation see as its priorities and essential to the business? (mandatory)

These answers are then brought together in the policy statement and the procedures and form the statutory and mandatory standards of good practice for the organisation.

Matching mandatory training requirements to organisational need

It is useful to consider this in a little more detail as establishing the mandatory requirements needs to be directly connected to the things that are essential for the organisation to achieve its objectives.

Following a simple checklist can enable an organisation to establish what it considers to be its mandatory training. This will vary from organisation to organisation as priorities, culture and climates will vary.

A checklist for defining mandatory training requirements is included in Appendix 2.

- **Identify organisational priorities**. The organisation uses its identified priorities to set out an annual work programme. The workforce will require a set of knowledge and skills (a core skill set) to be able to deliver those priorities. Mandatory training should ensure that the workforce has the basic skill set to deliver the outcomes required.
- **Consider national targets**. Performance monitoring of public sector organisations may require the organisation to adapt its priorities to recognise some national/regional benchmark or target that its performance will be measured against, i.e. income and expenditure balance resulting in financial solvency. This may require a level of budgetary control or financial awareness throughout an organisation.

- **Define the skill set**. Establish the core skill set required to deliver organisational objectives, i.e. if an organisational objective is to ensure that every member of the workforce has an annual appraisal then line managers should have 'appraisal training' as mandatory for their level of responsibility and staff should have a session on 'getting the most from your annual appraisal', perhaps as part of the mandatory induction programme.
- **Agree and ratify mandatory training requirement**. The organisation will need to establish a process for compiling and ratifying mandatory training as an organisational standard. This may involve the chief executive or board formally agreeing to implement it through their normal channels. Other organisations may wish to consult with the workforce through staff forums or committees before formally adopting the process as an organisational standard.

Identifying the training needs of the workforce

Seeing statutory and mandatory training as necessary to develop core skills means that these basic and often generic subjects are not overlooked in the key planning processes used by the organisation. Making them integral to the corporate planning process ensures that:

- mandatory core skills training establishes competence (safety), capability (ability to manage change) and capacity (ability to deal with large and complex workloads) throughout the workforce
- the corporate planning process establishes the work programme for the coming year, identifying the absolute deliverables for achieving performance targets and objectives and highlighting the subsequent training needs associated with them

- the organisation, having identified the required training, includes a training budget in its running costs that finances the training requirement
- there is a corporate mechanism for identifying training needs which is usually linked with appraisal or personal development planning processes already in operation. Whatever the

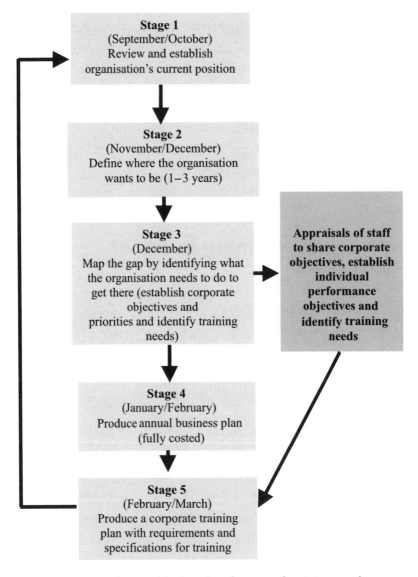

Figure 1.1   Harmonised timetable for identification of training needs.

mechanism, it needs to be responsive to the climate and culture of the organisation and the environment in which it operates.

The mechanism used to identify training needs has to be flexible enough to monitor the change agenda and ensure that staff are equipped to perform their duties in a timely fashion. Where timescales between corporate planning cycles and appraisals and training providers are not harmonised, the information detailing training need could be 12 months old before it is actioned. Figure 1.1 is a simple flowchart that offers an example of a harmonised timetable.

A harmonised approach ensures that the organisation is more accurately identifying training needs and can therefore commission training provision more effectively.

Using identified needs to commission effective training

By taking such a systematic approach to the identification of training needs, the organisation benefits from having more flexible provision which is cost efficient and practically effective.

Provision needs to be flexible in order to cater for the different levels of staff and equal access opportunities (location, time and method) and to be able to respond to organisational changes quickly.

Cost efficiency means analysing the statutory and mandatory training need to deliver the most effective training to the workforce as it needs it. Options may include:

- in-house training provision: sessions delivered by skilled (teaching) experts in the topic area, e.g. community practice tutors delivering manual handling or cross-infection training
- generic training programmes provided by similar or specialist organisations that share an understanding of the issues, e.g. a care home manager delivering training on medicines management in residential homes to local residential home staff

- practically effective statutory and mandatory training that delivers increased knowledge, skills development and individuals making competent judgements.

Staff involvement is important at this stage to ensure their support of the needs analysis process and to enable accurate assessment of requirement (regardless of their level in the organisation), giving a clear picture of perceived need. Their support is also needed for the organisation's risk assessment process to make sure that actual needs identified through error, omissions, complaints or problems are accommodated within statutory and mandatory training. This can only be achieved with a workforce that understands that risk management mechanisms are about learning and identification of training need and not about blame and retribution.

Clarifying statutory and mandatory training which is role specific requires the involvement of the line manager and post holder to agree the level and range of mandatory training required. A process similar to job evaluation is carried out where the role is broken down into core skills and knowledge and compared to the organisation's standard. A straightforward crossmatching takes place to identify the elements of mandatory training that apply to the role. These elements are added to any statutory training and professional competence-related training already identified.

NHS organisations

For NHS organisations (acute trusts, primary care trusts, walk-in centres, general practices, dentists, opticians, pharmacists, etc.) it is important to note key policy changes nationally that may impact on the organisation's statutory and mandatory training requirements. Examples of this may include:

- raised security status of public buildings
- Agenda for Change
- Knowledge and Skills Framework.

Raised security status of public buildings

Issues of security are a priority for public sector organisations in the current climate and it is important that organisations treat these issues seriously and plan for them. Regular security and evacuation drills may form part of an organisation's mandatory training if it is in a sensitive or vulnerable area.

Agenda for Change

This is the new NHS pay system that harmonises conditions of service across the wide range of disciplines. The new system is intended to offer a more transparent reward system for flexible working and to implement a structured approach to role redesign.

The Changing Workforce Programme is a national initiative intended to create the right educational, legal and regulatory framework to enable role redesign. Any significant changes to roles may impact the statutory and mandatory training requirement.

Knowledge and Skills Framework (KSF)

The KSF is an NHS staff development tool that:

- identifies the skills and knowledge that individuals need to apply in their posts
- helps to guide the development of individuals
- provides a common framework on which to base the review and development of all NHS staff
- provides a basis for pay progression through the NHS.

The framework contains core skills that the NHS considers to be part of the base skill set for all employees. Therefore, they will be adopted by all NHS employing organisations and will have an impact on the statutory and mandatory training requirement.

Requirements of the healthcare professions

Each professional body will have specific requirements for their members that are linked to their code of practice, their professional competence and accountability or their continuing professional development (CPD).

The organisation knows the skill mix of its workforce and the professions represented within it. It is important that it formally acknowledges those professional requirements and integrates them into role-specific statutory and mandatory training. Although many organisations expect individual professionals to keep up to date with this information and maintain records of their statutory and mandatory training status, this should be supported by responsible employers providing appropriate mechanisms and communication to make it as easy as possible.

Social care organisations

Professional social workers and those supporting social care generally are governed by a code of ethics for social work. This contains a comprehensive view of the values, principles and core behaviours essential to ethical social care. This is a vital document to shape the mandatory training requirements of those workers it covers.

Section 2:

Ensuring a robust infrastructure for statutory and mandatory training

Developing processes

Risk assessment processes are key elements in maintaining an organisation's legal compliance with regulations and minimising the risks affecting it. They can apply to physical, financial, service, clinical/care and business risks and should feed any skill gaps or procedural omissions identified into effective statutory and mandatory training programmes. Some common risk assessment tools that organisations use include:

- significant event analysis or critical incident analysis (*see* Appendix 5)
- risk assessment activity linked to health & safety (*see* Appendix 6)
- root cause analysis
- supervision/clinical supervision
- regulation/inspection visits
- clinical governance activity.

Practical identification of training needs

The corporate planning process is the first link in the chain of determining training needs. It is a cycle of activities that systematically identifies what needs to be done to move an organisation from its current position to where it needs to be in the future. It establishes a logical order to identifying training needs as well as a way of discovering problems and potential solutions. It also establishes an effective method for measuring achievements and outcomes.

The corporate planning cycle creates a context for identifying statutory and mandatory training needs by establishing a baseline of the current situation and a goal for where the endpoint will be. This enables the organisation to define the core skill and knowledge set needed to achieve the business objectives and performance standards it has established through the process.

Implementation of training is supported by clear stages for measuring need and setting objectives and a monitoring mechanism for spotting improvements and amendments to keep the organisation on track.

On an individual level the identification of training needs is part of the appraisal process. Employees will review their previous year's performance with their line manager/peer, consider the objectives for the coming year and identify what support/training they require to meet the organisation's standards. They will also review their training record to date and ensure that they have the required statutory and mandatory training set out by legislation and the organisation's own standards.

This information is then gathered together from individual members of the workforce and used to develop a corporate training

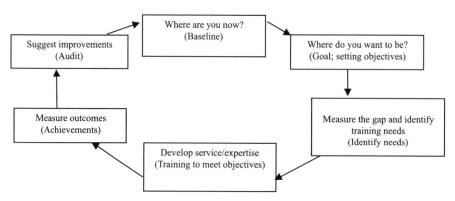

Figure 2.1   The corporate planning process.

plan. This record reflects all the statutory, mandatory, professional and personal development training required by the organisation in the coming year. It is then fed back into the corporate planning process to ensure that the plan has resources allocated and the training can be effectively commissioned.

Five basic steps to needs analysis

- **Step 1**. Collect information on current position by interviewing and discussing with all relevant individuals, internal and external. Define where the organisation wants to be.
- **Step 2**. Set objectives, targets and standards required (based on the information from step 1).
- **Step 3**. Identify the core skills and knowledge set required to deliver organisational objectives.
- **Step 4**. Compare this information with the identified training needs from staff appraisals.
- **Step 5**. Allocate resources and commission statutory and mandatory training by critically evaluating existing provision against the organisation's definitions and standards.

Measuring competence

Statutory and mandatory training is important to the organisation and yet, traditionally, it is an area where there is little requirement to prove competence. By building a competence measure into statutory and mandatory training, the organisation is setting a standard of safe and competent practice and could provide evidence of that if required to do so.

Testing competence requires more than attendance at an event but it should not be an onerous procedure. There should be a variety of methods in place for testing competence to ensure that staff attending statutory/mandatory training are absorbing it into their practice and not just hearing the information. Methods include the following.

- **Multiple-choice quiz (MCQ)**. Generally consists of a brief statement or problem (the stem) followed by a series of choices, of which one, all or some may be correct.
- **True/false questionnaires**.
- **Scenario questions**. Present a brief scenario, followed by one or more questions which are to be answered in an open-ended (if limited) fashion.
- **Oral tests**. Often begin with a case or scenario, asking the individual how he/she would manage it.
- **Testing skill**. Observed skill assessment with fixed and pre-tested set of physical manoeuvres to be performed, often on a mannequin or other patient simulator.
- **Testing attitude**. Using a global rating scale (e.g. Likert scale) to rate a series of statements expressing values, or beliefs, with which the individual may indicate strong agreement, agreement, disagreement, strong disagreement or a neutral response.
- **Standardised patients/clients**. Individuals trained to portray a set of clinical symptoms or care history and often able to elicit knowledge, skills and attitudes from the clinician/care professional being tested.

Each organisation should also have an evaluation policy and process in place to measure the effectiveness of learning undertaken by its staff. These results should form part of the individual's training record.

Monitoring status of statutory and mandatory training

Accurate records must be maintained that show who has received training and when. These are important data needed for corporate governance purposes or in the event of an incident that results in legal challenge. As a result, there is a need for organisations to monitor individual competence levels to confirm safe practice and to monitor reviews and updates to ensure compliance with the legislation.

- **Legal compliance**. Full and comprehensive records demonstrate organisational responsibility and compliance.
- **Professional compliance**. Up-to-date status of practising professionals, ensuring they are eligible and insurable to practise.

Developing a statutory and mandatory training policy

Organisations should issue a statutory/mandatory training policy (*see* Appendix 7) that includes:

- definitions of statutory and mandatory training
- statement of intent/organisational standards
- consequences of non-compliance
- explicit links to organisational procedures, e.g. clinical governance, risk management and HR policies
- explicit links to the organisation's business planning and workforce planning processes and learning strategy.

Compiling an organisational list of statutory/ mandatory training (see Appendix 4 for checklist)

The regulations for health & safety statutory training are clear:

> Employers have a duty under the Health & Safety at Work Act 1974 to take reasonable measures to ensure the health, safety and welfare of their employees at work. The also have a duty towards people who are not their employees but who use their premises.

Although the organisation has ultimate responsibility to make sure that this happens, everyone operating in the work environment has some responsibility for safety in the workplace by understanding safe practice, risk assessment and reporting. They need to check that their behaviour does not create risks and hazards and meets health, safety and welfare regulations.

Basic statutory training requirements include:

- familiarisation with the health & safety regulations and measures taken by the organisation to create and maintain a safe work environment (given initially when an employee first starts working for the organisation, usually forming part of the induction programme)
- nominated first aiders (for organisations employing more than five members of staff, the ratio is one first aider to every 25 employees and certification renewal is required every three years)
- annual fire safety training to ensure prevention and evacuation procedures are understood and adhered to (with nominated fire marshals to conduct safe evacuation of premises).

There are others but these are role specific and may not apply to everyone in the organisation, e.g. manual handling training for those working with loads or whose job requires them to lift.

The organisation should map its workforce in terms of roles and responsibilities and cross-reference them against statutory requirements to ensure it has adequate provision for its workforce.

Setting up a policy

Your organisation will probably want to have a policy that sets out its approach to statutory and mandatory training. By doing this you can, in a consistent and clear way:

- place statutory and mandatory training in the appropriate context

- state clearly what the organisation regards as statutory and mandatory training
- establish how decisions will be made in the future about what statutory and mandatory training exists
- set out the obligations of everyone involved
- describe a process for dealing with any issues or queries.

In order to place statutory and mandatory training in the appropriate context, the organisation needs to have a robust risk assessment process in place for hazards relating to the working environment and the practices and operations conducted in the normal course of business.

It might be considered good practice to have an overall training and development policy rather than one solely for statutory and mandatory training. The advantage of this approach is that it presents a holistic view of training, avoiding a clear division between that which we must do and that which we want to do.

The policy needs to include:

- organisational responsibilities – to staff, service users and the public – and which aspects of statutory and mandatory training are indicated by the nature of the business
- references to any training or learning strategies that the organisation operates to ensure a holistic approach to healthy and safe working
- references to specific frameworks, regulations or operational guidelines that the organisation has to adhere to, e.g. clinical and corporate governance for health organisations or CSCI regulations for care homes
- any special aims of the organisation that achieving excellence in this area might contribute to.

The organisation must publish a list of what it regards as statutory and mandatory training for its workforce. Having this captured in a document is very valuable, especially if it is kept electronically and is easily updated.

It is potentially dangerous to have various directorates or departments within an organisation making unilateral decisions or assumptions because no central guidance is easily available. Inconsistencies can result that may undermine the way the organisation's approach to statutory and mandatory training is perceived, both internally and externally.

It gives both the organisation and staff security to know that if they download guidance from an organisation's intranet/website, it will be up to date and they can rely on it. This might include:

- the ratified definitions of what constitutes statutory and mandatory training
- matrices or lists of specific role requirements.

Once a matrix exists of what is statutory and mandatory and its application to roles, it will need to be reviewed and updated annually to ensure it remains current. Having the process set out in a policy, especially if the period between reviews is also set out, will help achieve consistency. If staff change or the organisational structure changes there will still be no doubt that a certain process should be followed and it is not appropriate to take an *ad hoc* approach to such a fundamental issue. This might include:

- a step-by-step process to suggest a change and have it approved; this can be as simple or complex as is appropriate
- some things that may result in a need to change the matrix to give guidance, such as a change in the law on health & safety or the results of an organisational audit, review or inspection.

Setting out the obligations of everyone involved helps to reinforce responsibilities. As well as managers and directors being clear about what they must do, it will ensure that staff feel able to take a proactive approach. If someone is not getting what they need because another party has omitted to do something they should, such a statement can empower them to ask for it where they may not have felt able to before. In a complex and geographically dispersed organisation this is particularly useful. It may prevent a situation arising where no-one undertakes a task because everyone believes that someone else is doing it! Such a document might include:

- a list of obligations for every party, such as staff member, manager, directorate head, organisation, possibly an outsourcer or training department
- detail about how the obligations in other policies interact, such as the need for appraisal or clinical supervision
- clarification that processes like appraisal and compiling/ implementing a personal development plan are two-way. They are not procedures that are 'done to' staff; they should actively participate in them.

Defining the process for dealing with queries adds strength to a policy. People will have questions and problems, especially with a new policy, so it is useful to set out what to do if queries arise. This is not intended to usurp any other grievance or disciplinary procedure of the organisation; it is a way of tackling any glitches before they become serious problems. This might include:

- who to contact first of all
- a statement that if someone is not able to participate equitably then the organisation is committed to helping them do so
- possibly how a serious issue might escalate (maybe through the discipline and grievance procedure)
- some examples of problems that ought to be brought up if they arise.

Identifying training needs: the process

The identification of training needs can be a simple or complex process, depending on the desired outcome.

A comprehensive process may be what the organisation aspires to, but it may be limited by available resources (time and money).

The most direct and effective way is to build identification of training needs into the appraisal process. During the interview, ask the following questions.

- What is the statutory and mandatory training requirement for your role? This tests understanding and clarifies the requirement.
- How does your training record to date compare? This clarifies the current situation and highlights gaps in record keeping or access issues.
- What do you need to complete in the coming year to meet organisational and professional requirements? This identifies the statutory/mandatory training need for the coming year.

This process can also be extended to identify general training needs.

Quality criteria for selecting training providers

It can be useful to consider the quality standards the organisation requires when selecting effective training providers. These can be brought together in a simple 'shopping list' of criteria used in the selection or tendering process.

- Specialist training organisation with successful track record in the particular training area under consideration.
- Qualified trainers (specify a level of training qualification that engenders confidence in their professionalism, e.g. Chartered Institute of Personnel Development [CIPD] or similar).
- The training provider produces literature that contains:
  - course titles
  - aims and expected outcomes of the training
  - key learning objectives
  - target audience

- level of material (basic awareness, intermediate, advanced)
- competency measure
- method of evaluation
- training methods/learning style catered for
- award/verification/accreditation/affiliation.

Notes for NHS organisations

All employers have obligations toward their staff and customers to ensure that work takes place in a safe and competent manner. In the NHS these obligations take on particular importance.

Achieving this often means training staff. In the NHS the 'cost' of staff training (including the time spent away from the workplace undertaking training in terms of lost clinical sessions and so on) is felt as keenly as the material cost of funding a place on a course.

This toolkit is designed to help NHS organisations do two things:

- help them to identify who needs to do what training and how often
- enable them to think about ways to improve staff competence that do not involve spending time away from work repeating courses (where this is appropriate).

This is a practical resource that helps organisations to meet their obligations and provide supporting evidence of legal compliance with the minimum of bureaucracy, wasted time and effort.

Organisational obligations

In the NHS these obligations are especially complex, not least because they come from a variety of sources including:

- the law
- professional bodies

- governmental and quasi-governmental bodies
- internal policies and procedures
- meeting service needs
- common sense!

Why is this so important?

The sanction for failing to meet obligations varies from possible imprisonment (for example, should an employee be killed or badly injured in the course of their work through the organisation's negligence) through to patient complaints to be dealt with where services are poorly provided.

It is more productive to think of the benefits of getting this right than the consequences of things going wrong. Although the training dealt with in this toolkit is described as 'statutory and mandatory', the skills and knowledge covered are all practically useful. Thinking of statutory and mandatory training as a chore or formality undermines its value. We all need to know what to do in a fire; if we are required to practise the efficient evacuation of buildings, it is just as easy to take professional pride in doing it well.

Patient safety and risk management are key considerations for NHS trusts. By having a high-quality way of meeting statutory and mandatory training requirements, an NHS trust can begin to feel confident that it is addressing these key issues. However, by being able to demonstrate that its staff are competent, a trust is in a strong position to feel that it is minimising the risk of things going wrong.

Currently NHS organisations conduct training and assume competence of their staff through attendance. Very few measure the competence of their staff in statutory and mandatory training areas. By addressing statutory and mandatory training in a clear and consistent way an organisation can make the link between compliance and competence. This is beneficial to staff and the organisation as valuable resources will be used appropriately. Attention can then be turned to the broader (but no less important!) task of staff development.

Why is this difficult?

As an example, line managers have to ensure that everyone does know what to do in a fire. The potential pitfall is that they might send someone on a half-day fire course that has little relevance to their workplace. It may tell them the evacuation process of a multistorey hospital building when their environment is a multi-wing, single-storey community nursing unit.

This approach has led to many individuals attending annual refresher days and paying little attention as they have heard the same 'lecture' before and they feel it is too removed from their situation to be relevant.

The organisation also needs to develop a culture in which it is common practice to demonstrate the ability and competence to do things to the required standard of your role, whether it is using a computer or taking blood.

Statutory responsibility of NHS organisations

The modern NHS places staff and patients at the heart of healthcare provision. Achieving this means developing a front-line workforce able to use their skills and knowledge effectively in delivering efficient services in innovative ways. This demands a highly competent and educated workforce.

As NHS organisations need to provide a strategic framework to deliver these services, staff training will be a central focus to ensure services are delivered effectively and safely to patients. The foundation of this is meeting basic obligations – getting statutory and mandatory training right. While it is only the start of the process to develop staff so that they realise their potential, it is essential.

Setting standards

When considering statutory and mandatory training for staff, it is important to define exactly what standard of performance is required as an outcome of the training. Without this level of clarity it will be very difficult to know if the training meets the requirements of the organisation or to evaluate the effect on staff performance in the workplace.

This can be a difficult area to address. In respect of manual handling, for example, it is not sufficient to say that a competent member of staff is able to lift. When it comes to an individual it is necessary to consider what they will be required to lift and the circumstances in which they will do so, such as the environment and the height of the lift. A risk assessment would be a useful source of information to allow the organisation to define very clearly and in detail how it expects the task to be performed. This is important to enable people to recognise competence when they see it and, conversely, to know what areas need improvement when there is an issue.

Having these standards has many benefits.

- It means that staff can refer to them and refresh their memory.
- Good standards will mean that several people can use them to observe a staff member and assess their performance consistently.
- It helps in giving feedback – to describe how performance differed from what is required and explain what needs to be done differently to meet the standard.
- In the event of any disagreement about whether or not some-one is competent, it is easier to produce evidence on which to make a decision as long as the person making the original assessment kept factual notes of what they saw being done.
- In terms of training, the standards are the quality control criteria for any education offered. The outcome of the training will be a group of people who can perform the task to the specified standard.

Having a set of clear, detailed and unambiguous standards that define competent performance in the areas covered by statutory and mandatory training will give the organisation a solid base from which to demonstrate that risks are being effectively minimised.

Record keeping

Record keeping is critical. It is uncomfortable to be in a position where the organisation is unable to prove that it meets performance criteria, not because it has not provided the correct level of statutory and mandatory training but because the records giving evidence of such training do not exist.

A comprehensive database that captures the activity and status of individual staff members is ideal. A simple spreadsheet or paper record is harder to report from but will do the job.

Liability when things do go wrong

Things do go wrong. People make mistakes, equipment fails and things don't always go without a hitch.

As an employing organisation it is important to be in a position to show that everything that could be done to limit the risk of avoidable mistakes and accidents has been done. Risk management is a large topic and for the purposes of the toolkit, the focus is on the role of good practice in training (specifically, statutory and mandatory training) in managing risk. The organisation may want to link their statutory and mandatory training policy directly into their risk management process for clinical and corporate governance and other aspects of operational business. Failure to make explicit links may result in duplicating work or missing out key elements altogether.

The key to this approach is to ensure that statutory and mandatory training has been completed consistently and rigorously. This starts with being able to show the rationale for deciding what was statutory and mandatory and for whom. Minutes of decision-making meetings (disagreements as well as decisions made) will provide the organisation with a tangible record. They can also act as a valuable *aide-mémoire* when the policy on statutory and mandatory training is reviewed.

Producing a matrix of what is statutory and mandatory for the organisation and its varying professional/staff groups is a practical way of disseminating complex information (*see* Appendix 3). This, together with the minutes, provides an audit trail the organisation can use for internal purposes and they may be produced for Health Commission inspectors or the internal/external auditor when required. Nothing inspires confidence in the effectiveness of an organisation like being able to produce evidence of good practice in an organised way rather than trying to forensically reconstruct what happened from fragmented documentation and, even worse, memory.

Some useful tips

- If you are giving someone a booklet or policy to read and act on then get them to sign for it.
- If you are having real difficulty getting an individual or their manager to co-operate and undertake training, ensure they understand the consequences of their actions and compile a record of correspondence summarising conversations, requests, dates and times. If there is a resulting disciplinary action or problem, this will provide evidence of their negligence to act appropriately.
- At training courses, have registers that you have pre-printed with names to sign next to. Signatures alone are difficult to decipher.

Being able to show that you have taken a thoughtful and appropriate approach to staff training will make it easier to prove that the organisation did all it could to prevent the incident occurring. This is obviously broader than meeting statutory and mandatory training requirements – we all have skills and knowledge necessary to do our job that are neither statutory nor mandatory. Showing that statutory and mandatory training is up to date will be a good start. Being able to show that all staff have personal development plans and a record of their training would be even better!

If things go wrong because an NHS organisation or one of its employees has been negligent, the injured party can take legal action for damages, e.g. this may be another employee or visitor to an NHS building who falls over a pile of boxes carelessly left in a corridor. In a situation like this, the NHS organisation will need to consider if it can provide evidence that the person who left the boxes there had been told that it was not acceptable. This will mean proving that the individual had been trained to know the health & safety standards they were expected to meet and that it was not custom and practice to leave boxes in corridors. The NHS organisation will want to prevent this happening by making sure that its staff are up to date with current good practice.

Organisational versus personal responsibility

Statutory and mandatory training can only work coherently if the organisation and staff work together. Responsibility for getting it right is shared between the organisation, managers and the staff members undertaking the training. When problems occur it may be a result of complex workloads, conflicting priorities or short deadlines. Often it is due to other things being perceived as higher priority.

Infrastructure

NHS organisations have to make sure that everything is in place to enable their staff to meet their obligations. This will start with identifying what is statutory and mandatory and for whom. You then have to make sure that this information is readily available and known to be so. You next have to provide the training itself. In an NHS organisation this will involve making sure that the training is available in a format that suits all staff (such as those with unusual working patterns, sited at remote locations or working in the community). The organisation needs to carefully consider the specific circumstances and needs of its workforce in order to achieve this.

The role of record keeping will ultimately fall to the organisation as the commissioner and/or provider. Accurate records for each training event need to be maintained on a spreadsheet or manually, whichever is easier. Basic information should include:

- a list of who is registered to attend a programme
- an attendance register with signatures
- a list of those who cancelled or failed to attend on the day
- the evaluation report on the outcomes and learning experience from attending delegates.

If the organisation has commissioned the training from an external provider it may be useful to keep more detailed records for audit purposes. These could contain:

- any decision-making paperwork about why the provider was selected
- copies of the programme
- a set of course materials
- financial records of contracts, payments, etc.

There is an important role for quality control in this process. Did the training meet the need it was intended to meet? The organisation needs to know this to be able to demonstrate a return on investment. At the beginning of the commissioning process, what evidence would there need to be to demonstrate that the organisation's criteria or standards had been met? A planned evaluation would identify these key outcomes. This involves following up delegates and their line managers to ascertain what attending delegates have done differently as a result of the training (how has their practice changed/improved?).

NHS managers

Managers have a responsibility to ensure that statutory and mandatory training is effective as they know in the greatest detail who requires what training within their team/department. They need to keep accurate records of what has been done, what needs to be done and review dates for updating statutory and mandatory training. It is this information that will enable their organisation to plan training provision appropriately.

Managers also have to take an active role in getting staff through the necessary training. In an environment where staffing levels are tight it is often difficult to release staff to train. Unexpected events mean that cancellations may occur at short notice. It is important to remember that time spent meeting statutory and mandatory training requirements is work. It should be planned into work time and treated in the same way as other routine tasks. If it is put off repeatedly then a backlog will develop which will inevitably mean it becomes impossible to release several staff for time to catch up on training they could have been doing over a longer period.

Managing statutory and mandatory training (and other staff development) is part of the manager's job. If staff are not able to do it then there is a problem that the manager needs to address and an organisational risk developing. It may also signify a training need of the manager concerned.

The NHS organisation has a role to play in supporting this. When planning training timetables, it is important to ensure that subjects are staggered throughout the year. If a single training topic takes place in 'clusters', it becomes more difficult for all relevant staff to leave their work base to attend the training in rapid succession.

NHS staff

Staff members have a responsibility to undertake statutory and mandatory training to ensure they are safe and competent to do their job. This begins by checking that they are aware of what is statutory and mandatory for their role. If this is unclear, the exact details should be sought from the line manager or training department (if the organisation has one).

The individual is ultimately responsible for undertaking the training and should take this seriously, giving it appropriate priority. Individuals should not wait to be chased or reminded and this applies equally to staff members who have a professional body to report to and support workers who do not. It can be useful for the individual to keep a personal record of completed training as part of their personal development plan, along with any certificates, reflective journal entries and review dates.

If there are problems finding time to complete statutory and mandatory training or in accessing courses, the issue should be raised with the line manager.

It is then up to the individual to take the opportunity and use what has been learnt back in the workplace. Statutory and mandatory training is not a hoop to be jumped through; it is done because there is a need to know or review what it covers. There should also be an opportunity to give feedback at the end of a course: to comment on the content, omissions, etc. and to offer suggestions on how it could be improved.

Section 3:

Training programme outlines

The following suggested outlines offer:

- a rationale for the training
- target groups the session may apply to
- frequency of update
- key content
- suggested methods of delivery
- suggested competence measures.

They are intended as a guide only. They need to be measured against the roles and responsibilities of the target group within the organisation and adjusted accordingly.

The organisation's own core skill set will also influence training session content.

General health & safety induction training: S001

Rationale
The organisation is required by law to ensure that all its employees receive information relevant to their (and others including the public) health, safety and well-being related to or at their work. The organisation is also required to ensure that all employees are aware of their responsibilities and procedures to assess and manage all clinical and other types of risks and report things when they go wrong. Information provided will be general rather than role specific and therefore relevant to all new employees, to provide sufficient information early in employment to work safely. This will not negate the need for more intensive training to meet the needs of specific roles and/or responsibilities.

Staff Group
All new employees.

Frequency
New employees should attend as soon as possible and no later than six weeks after starting employment.

Topics
- General health & safety at work
- Legal background
- Principles of risk assessment and management
- Accident and incident reporting
- Fire safety – prevention and actions in the event of an emergency
- Personal safety, lone working, violence and aggression, zero tolerance

- Infection control policy and procedures
- Handwashing/hand hygiene
- Principles of manual handling and safe load movement
- Occupational health services, including HIV awareness
- Infection control, including needlestick injuries and waste management
- Environmental issues
- Organisation's policies

Suggested Methods of Delivery
One-day programme to be delivered twice monthly.
Co-ordinated by the health & safety adviser with input from colleagues knowledgeable on specific subjects.
Courses advertised through in-house training prospectus.

Suggested Competence Measures
Question and answer.
Oral questioning.

Departmental/role-specific health & safety instruction: S002

Rationale
The Management of Health & Safety at Work Regulations 1999 and Clinical Negligence Standards state that every manager has responsibility for ensuring staff are provided with the correct information and instruction to work safely and for ongoing supervision that health and safety procedures are followed and any safety equipment policies and guidance provided are correctly utilised.

The manager must establish, in discussion with new employees, the essential health & safety information relevant to the post. They must verify whether the employee has sufficient existing knowledge through previous training and/or experience to work safely (preferably with documentary evidence) and make arrangements for any shortfalls to be addressed.

Staff Group
All new employees.

Frequency
On commencement of employment prior to carrying out duties of the post and then reviewed at least annually.

Topics
This will vary according to need and risk assessment. However, it is expected the following will be required as a minimum for all new employees on commencement.

- Clinical risk assessment and management procedures, e.g. care co-ordination

- Fire exits, evacuation procedures and assembly point. Any specific fire hazards
- Identify hazards within workplace and provide instruction on how to work safely
- VDU assessment
- Electrical equipment testing
- Instruction on use of safety equipment and safe use of equipment routinely used
- Security issues

Specific topics may include: use of display screen equipment, COSHH, radiation protection.

Suggested Methods of Delivery
Instruction to be carried out at the place of work by the individual's manager or nominated representative/s, e.g. a suitably experienced/trained/qualified member of staff.
Staff induction pack.

Suggested Competence Measures
Question and answer.
Oral test.

COSHH: S003

Rationale
This is a basic introduction to the Control of Substances Hazardous to Health (COSHH) Regulations 2002 to raise awareness of the issues and the policies put in place by the organisation to minimise the risks.

Staff Group
All employees, temporary/bank staff and subcontractors.

Frequency
One off.

Topics
- Overview of COSHH regulations
- Understand when the regulations apply
- Understand how to operate safely in an environment containing hazardous substances

Suggested Methods of Delivery
E-learning.
In-house session.
Part of a comprehensive health & safety programme.

Suggested Competence Measures
Question and answer.
Multiple-choice paper.
Observation.

RIDDOR: S004

Rationale
This session is an introduction to the Reporting of Injuries, Diseases and Dangerous Occurrences Regulations 1995 to raise awareness of policies and procedures put in place by the organisation.

Staff Group
All employees, temporary/bank staff and subcontractors.

Frequency
One off.

Topics
- Overview of RIDDOR regulations
- Understand when the regulations apply
- Understand the reporting process and implications of non-compliance

Suggested Methods of Delivery
E-learning.
In-house session.
Part of a comprehensive health & safety programme.

Suggested Competence Measures
Question and answer.
Multiple-choice paper.
Observation.

Fire safety sessions/updates: S005

Rationale
All organisations are required to conduct fire safety training for their employees that covers safety, prevention and evacuation procedures as a duty under the Health & Safety at Work Act 1974. In addition, the NHS Act states that all NHS employees must receive training in fire safety, prevention and evacuation procedures.

Staff Group
All employees.

Frequency
Annual update for general information and fire safety awareness.

Topics
- Fire prevention and safety
- Evacuation procedures

Suggested Methods of Delivery
Fire lectures.
Local specific training by fire safety officer.
E-learning module.

Suggested Competence Measures
Question and answer.
Multiple-choice paper.
Observation.

Workplace risk assessment: S006

Rationale
The Management of Health & Safety at Work Regulations 1999 state that every manager has responsibility for ensuring staff are provided with the correct information and instruction to work safely, and for ongoing supervision that health and safety procedures are followed and any safety equipment provided is correctly utilised. This requires managers to have a good understanding of their responsibilities for health & safety and to be competent in carrying out workplace risk assessments. This is also a requirement under the NHS Clinical Negligence and Controls Assurance processes as part of the core risk management standards.

Staff Group
All managers with risk assessment responsibilities, i.e. all operational line managers who supervise people, activities and/or premises for both clinical and non-clinical staff. Employees with delegated responsibility to undertake workplace risk assessments.

Frequency
On commencement in post and updated every three years.

Cont.

Topics

Responsibilities for risk assessment at work

- Legal background
- Identifying workplace hazards
- Determining and prioritising levels of risk
- Managing and minimising risk
- Developing risk control strategies and implementing risk treatment plans
- Developing departmental risk registers
- Accident and incident prevention and investigation
- Record keeping and documentation

Basic health & safety information to improve understanding of specific topics relevant to place of work, e.g.:

- COSHH
- Use of display screen equipment
- Fire safety
- Electrical safety
- Radiation
- First aid
- Manual handling
- Personal protective equipment/infection control
- Provision and use of work equipment
- Workplace regulations
- Medical equipment
- Violence and aggression
- Employment of young people
- Expectant mothers
- Vulnerable groups

Suggested Methods of Delivery

Courses will be advertised through in-house training prospectus and flyers.
External programme.

Suggested Competence Measure

Accredited test.

Manual handling – back awareness: S007A

Rationale

The Manual Handling Operations Regulations 1992 require all employees to be aware of and use safe manual handling practices in the workplace.

Many staff in non-clinical roles do not undertake significant load handling as part of their normal duties. The risks to this group of staff are therefore relatively low and it should be sufficient to provide information on the principles of safe load movement and back care.

Where the job role involves significant load handling, then 'key workers' should be nominated who can undertake risk assessments in conjunction with the line manager and deliver specific training as required.

Staff Group

All non-clinical staff that undertake moving and handling of loads as part of their duties.

Clinical staff not involved in the moving and handling of patients.

Frequency

On commencement of employment and an update every two years.

Topics
- Principles of back care
- Principles and demonstration of safe movement and handling practices
- Risk assessment

Cont.

Suggested Method of Delivery
Courses advertised through in-house training prospectus and flyers.

Suggested Competence Measures
Observation of lift.
Question and answer.

Manual handling – patients: S007B

Rationale
The Manual Handling Operations Regulations 1992 require all employers to provide training for their employees in safe manual handling techniques and, most importantly, for the assessment and supervision of safe manual handling practices in the workplace. Significant costs of absence and compensation may result from back injury to healthcare workers.

Staff Group
All clinical and support staff involved in the moving and handling of patients.

Frequency
On commencement and an annual update.

Topics
- Principles of safe handling and movement:
  - overview of current legislation
  - injuries and statistics
  - anatomy and physiology of the back
  - causes of injury
- Best practice in patient handling techniques
- Use of equipment, hoists, etc.
- Risk assessment

Suggested Method of Delivery
Courses advertised through in-house training prospectus and flyers.

Suggested Competence Measures
Observation of lift.
Question and answer.

Infection control/sharps: S008

Rationale
To enable staff to protect themselves against injury and infection when handling sharps and to promote evidence-based standards of care in line with organisational policy.

Staff Group
All clinical and care staff.
All domestic staff.

Frequency
On commencement of employment via general health & safety induction programme.
Annual update.

Topics
Clinical staff
- Practical awareness of infection control
- Infections in the new millennium
- Infection control in clinical practice
- Audit – underpinning clinical governance
- Controls assurance – the government agenda

Non-clinical staff
- Hand washing
- Universal precautions
- Environment
- Sharps injury reporting
- Clinical waste

Suggested Methods of Delivery
Minimum two-hour sessions for non-clinical staff.
Large group update sessions and locally delivered tailored sessions for clinical staff.

All training could be delivered in house by the infection control nurse specialist.

Suggested Competence Measures
Question and answer.
Observation.

Cardiopulmonary resuscitation/ anaphylaxis: S009

Rationale
To promote a controlled response by healthcare workers faced with a case of anaphylaxis or heart failure.

Staff Group
All clinical staff.

Frequency
Annually.

Topics
- Issues concerning anaphylaxis
- Anaphylaxis packs
- First response
- Cardiopulmonary resuscitation skills

Suggested Methods of Delivery
Courses advertised through in-house training prospectus and flyers.
Training could take place within teams at the workplace.

Suggested Competence Measures
Question and answer.
Observation.

First aid: S010

Rationale
Health & safety regulations require all organisations with more than 20 employees to have a designated first aider, as good practice.

Staff Group
Members of staff nominated as 'first aider' or 'appointed person' (as a requirement of workplace risk assessments being undertaken).

Frequency
Prior to taking up responsibility and updated every three years.

Topics

First aider training
- HSE approved – three-day First Aid at Work course (valid for three years)
- HSE approved – two-day First Aid at Work requalification course
- (required prior to expiry of certificate)

Appointed person training
- Four-hour Emergency First Aid course, covering:
  - actions in an emergency
  - CPR
  - first aid for unconscious casualty
  - first aid for bleeding or wounded

Suggested Method of Delivery
External approved courses or via qualified first aid trainer, occupational health services.

Suggested Competence Measures
Assessed/validated test.
Observation.

Food hygiene: S011

Rationale
The 1995 Food Regulations state that all those involved in handling food should be trained appropriately.

Staff Group
Basic level − all staff who are involved in the preparation and serving of food to patients, services users, visitors and staff, e.g. catering staff, ward-based domestic staff, nursing staff, healthcare support staff, occupational therapists, certain speech and language therapists, dieticians.
Intermediate level − supervisory staff in portering, catering and housekeeping.
Advanced level − senior managers in catering and house-keeping.

Frequency
All levels − within 3−6 months of commencement in post with an update/refresher every three years.

Topics
- Bacteriology
- Personal hygiene
- Physical and bacterial contamination of food
- Food storage
- Cleaning and disinfection

Suggested Method of Delivery
External course via local/other provider.

Suggested Competence Measures
Question paper.
Observation.

Confidentiality, Caldicott Regulations and complaints: S012

Rationale
To ensure that all staff members are familiar with Caldicott Regulations governing confidentiality and the organisation's confidentiality and complaints policies.

Staff Group
All staff.

Frequency
One off.

Topics
- Caldicott Regulations and Guardians
- Confidentiality policy
- Obtaining consent (legalities and practice)
- Complaints process
- Patient Advice and Liaison Service (PALS)

Suggested Method of Delivery
In-house session by experienced staff member.

Suggested Competence Measures
Question paper.
Question and answer.

Data security and confidentiality: SO13

Rationale
The Data Protection Act 1998, controls assurance and clinical negligence standards require that all records are managed and controlled in such a way as to support safe practice, confidentiality and efficient operation of services in health and care settings.

Staff Group
All staff who are involved in the preparation and management of administrative and clinical/care records.

Frequency
This will vary according to need and risk assessment but should be completed within 3–6 months of commencement in post with an update/refresher following any major changes to requirements.

Topics
- Data Protection Act overview
- The completion, use, storage and retrieval of all health records pertaining to each patient, including giving patients or others access
- Developing a unified health record, which all professions use
- Filing and storage of patient records so that loss of documents and traces are minimised
- Readily identifiable notes on key treatments within patient's health records
- Storing and mounting test results (e.g. bloods, scans, X-rays) within patient's health records
- Computer systems, or other, for identifying and retrieving notes

- Arrangements for retrieval of notes from storage 24 hours a day, seven days a week
- Audit of record-keeping standards within team or professional group
- Arrangement for identifying records that must not be destroyed
- Confidentiality and 'ownership'
- Security and controlling access

Suggested Method of Delivery
In-house training sessions by specialist.

Suggested Competence Measures
Question and answer.
In-tray exercise.

Equality and diversity: SO14

Rationale
To develop the knowledge and skills of all staff managers, supervisors and team leaders about equality and diversity and the NHS Framework (or equivalent) and legal implications, with an overall objective of positively influencing recruitment and retention and improving working relationships.

Employment legislation requires employers to prevent discrimination at work and to promote racial equality. It is also a requirement in line with organisational policy.

Staff Group
All staff.

Frequency
As and when the policy is updated and/or amended.
A refresher for all newly appointed supervisors, managers, team leaders.

Topics
- The legal framework
- Policy, roles and responsibilities
- Recognising equality, diversity, harassment and bullying issues
- Dealing with and resolving concerns

Suggested Method of Delivery
In-house programme delivered using organisational policy and procedure and advertised through the training prospectus.

Suggested Competence Measures
Question and answer.
Scenarios.

Whistleblowing and fraud: S015

Rationale
To develop the knowledge and skills of all staff managers, supervisors and team leaders about the policy relating to public interest disclosure and the NHS (or equivalent) policy on fraud.

Staff Group
All staff.

Frequency
As and when the policy is updated and/or amended.
A refresher for all newly appointed managers, supervisors and team leaders.

Topic
● Key points of the policy and procedure

Suggested Method of Delivery
In-house programme delivered using organisational policy and procedure and advertised through the training prospectus.

Suggested Competence Measure
Question and answer.

Child protection: S016/017/018

Rationale

This training is a legal requirement for staff working with children and gives them an overview of the role of the area child protection committee (ACPC) and a better understanding of the categories of abuse. The training would help those directly working with children to consider the necessary action they would take in the event of a child protection concern and to understand their accountability and responsibility in relation to child protection.

Staff Group

All those with responsibility for providing a service to children need Level 1, at their manager's discretion.

Other staff, e.g. health visitors, midwives, paediatric nurses, practice nurses, healthcare assistants, carers, counsellors, etc.

Frequency

Introduction of Child Protection Level 1 – within three months of commencement.

Introduction to Working Together to Safeguard Children Level 2 – within one year of commencement.

Level 3 – every three years.

Topic

Refer to up-to-date content in ACPC training brochure.

Suggested Methods of Delivery

Level 1 – ACPC recommended half-day workshop in house: S016.

Level 2 – ACPC training brochure: S017.

Level 3 – ACPC training brochure: S018.

Suggested Competence Measure

Accredited test.

Major incident planning: S019

Rationale
Clinical negligence standards state that all employees with responsibility in these areas should be trained appropriately.

Staff Group
All qualified clinical staff who are involved in assessing and managing clinical risk, clinical adverse events, information to patients about interventions and treatments and obtaining consent, e.g. medical and nursing staff, occupational therapists, certain speech and language therapists, dieticians, dentists, psychologists.

Frequency
This will vary according to need and risk assessment but should be completed within three months of commencement in post with an update/refresher following any major changes to requirements.

Topics
- Clinical risk assessment and management and related policy and procedures, e.g. discharge planning
- The protection of the public and service users versus positive risk taking
- Assessment of patients for the possibility of self-harm or harm to others
- Managing the risk of self-harm or harm to others by service users
- Accessing and giving information about interventions to patients, including the risks and benefits
- Capability, consent and specific procedures, e.g. medicines
- Clinical adverse events, e.g. drug errors
- Disseminating and learning the lessons and acting on these

Cont.

- Informing patients when an adverse event occurs that involves them
- Informing carers and/or relatives when an adverse event occurs involving their loved one

Suggested Method of Delivery
Internal or multiagency courses advertised through training prospectus.

Suggested Competence Measure
Accredited test.

Electrical testing: S020

Rationale
To ensure that staff working with electrical equipment understand safe practice procedures.

Staff Group
All staff.

Frequency
One off.

Topics
- Electrical equipment covered
- Basic safety
- Reporting problems and risks

Suggested Method of Delivery
Workplace-based briefing session.

Suggested Competence Measure
Question and answer.

VDU assessment: S021

Rationale
To give an overview of the Display Screen Equipment Regulations 2002 governing working with VDUs and assessment processes.

Staff Group
All staff working with VDU equipment.

Frequency
One off.

Topics
- Assessing risk
- Promoting good practice
- Workplace design
- Operation times
- Pregnancy and working with VDUs

Suggested Method of Delivery
Workplace-based briefing session.

Suggested Competence Measure
Question and answer.

Waste management: S022

Rationale
An overview of specific waste management procedures to ensure compliance with COSHH Regulations.

Staff Group
All staff who come into contact with waste management.

Frequency
One off.

Topics
- Different waste products
- Clean-up procedures and equipment
- Cross-infection risk
- Waste management – coloured sacks
- Duty to dispose of waste
- Disposing of contaminated or confidential waste

Suggested Method of Delivery
Internal session delivered by specialist.

Suggested Competence Measure
Question and answer.

General induction: M001

Rationale
A process whereby new employees acclimatise to their job through an orientation course. This acts as a formal welcome to the organisation, providing an opportunity to inform new staff of some of the key issues of importance in relation to their roles and responsibilities.

Staff Group
All new employees.

Frequency
New employees should attend as soon as possible and no later than four weeks after starting employment.

Topics
- The organisation and the environment they operate in
- Structure of the organisation
- Values and principles of the organisation
- Customer care and complaints
- Confidentiality
- Knowledge management
- Clinical governance
- Wages, payroll and pensions
- Equality and diversity
- Employee rights and responsibilities
- Personal development

Suggested Method of Delivery
In-house session.

Suggested Competence Measure
Question and answer.

Departmental induction: M002

Rationale
A process whereby new employees, regardless of whether new to the organisation or an internal change, acclimatise to their job through socialisation, enabling them to build up working relationships and their roles within their new team. A local induction should be seen as an investment in an employee's growth, development and output, and in the organisation's efficiency, productivity and future success.

Staff Group
All new employees.

Frequency
New employees should have a departmental induction over their first eight weeks in their new role.

Topics
- Introductions to work colleagues
- Confirmation of post, hours, pay, etc.
- Completion of any forms and validity of registration documents, e.g. commencement form, qualifications, PIN, NI number
- Location of facilities
- Policies and procedures
- Local health & safety issues and risk assessment
- Identification of training

Suggested Method of Delivery
To be co-ordinated by the manager/supervisor/team leader of the department.

Suggested Competence Measure
Oral test.

Handling discipline at work: M003

Rationale
To develop the knowledge and skills of managers, supervisors and team leaders to deal effectively with issues relating to discipline at work, with an overall objective of improving and maintaining performance and understanding and observing the rules of natural justice.

Staff Group
All staff who have responsibility for managing others, particularly newly appointed supervisors, managers, team leaders.

Frequency
As and when the policy is updated and/or amended.

Topics
- The legal framework
- Organisation policy and procedure
- Roles and responsibilities
- Investigation
- Interviewing skills

Suggested Method of Delivery
In-house programme delivered using organisational policy and procedure and advertised through the training prospectus.

Suggested Competence Measures
Question and answer.
Role play.

Grievance and disputes: M004

Rationale
To develop the knowledge and skills of managers, supervisors and team leaders to deal effectively with grievances and disputes, with an overall objective of improving and maintaining performance and understanding and observing the rules of natural justice.

Staff Group
All staff who have responsibility for managing others, particularly newly appointed supervisors, managers, team leaders.

Frequency
As and when the policy is updated and/or amended.

Topics
- Definitions of grievances and disputes
- Aims and basic principles of the policy and procedure
- Stages of the procedure

Suggested Method of Delivery
In-house programme delivered using organisational policy and procedure and advertised through the training prospectus.

Suggested Competence Measures
Question and answer.
Role play.

Managing attendance: M005

Rationale
To develop the knowledge and skills of managers, supervisors and team leaders to deal effectively with managing attendance, with an overall objective of reducing absence and ensuring the organisational targets are met.

Employment legislation and ACAS codes of practice reinforce the need to train managers in the use of fair procedures for dealing with poor attendance and sickness absence. It is also a requirement in line with organisational policy.

Staff Group
All staff who have responsibility for managing others, particularly newly appointed supervisors, managers, team leaders.

Frequency
As and when the policy is updated and/or amended.

Topics
- Responsibility for managing attendance
- Policy
- Legislative context
- Managing return to work

Suggested Method of Delivery
In-house programme delivered using organisational policy and procedure and advertised through the training prospectus.

Suggested Competence Measures
Question and answer.
Role play.

Harassment and bullying: M006

Rationale
To develop the knowledge and skills of all staff managers, supervisors and team leaders about equality and diversity and the NHS Framework (or equivalent) and legal implications, with an overall objective of positively influencing recruitment and retention and improving working relationships.

Employment legislation requires employers to prevent discrimination at work and to promote racial equality. Health & safety legislation requires employers to provide a healthy and safe work environment. It is also a requirement in line with organisational policy.

Staff Group
All staff and a refresher for all newly appointed supervisors, managers, team leaders.

Frequency
As and when the policy is updated and/or amended.

Topics
- The legal framework
- Policy, roles and responsibilities
- Recognising equality, diversity, harassment and bullying issues
- Dealing with and resolving concerns

Suggested Method of Delivery
In-house programme delivered using organisational policy and procedure and advertised through the training prospectus.

Suggested Competence Measures
Question and answer.
Role play.

Recruitment interviewing skills: M007A

Rationale
For staff involved in the recruitment and selection process to develop first-hand experience in a safe environment, reducing the pitfalls and poor practice that could result in a financial implication for the organisation. Employment legislation and ACAS codes of practice reinforce the need to train managers in the use of fair procedures for recruiting new staff and to prevent discrimination in selection procedures. The selection interview is the most common form of recruitment used and potentially the most subjective part of the process.

Staff Group
All staff who have responsibility for recruitment and selection in their work area, in particular all newly appointed staff with responsibility for recruitment and selection.

Frequency
As and when the policy is updated and/or amended.

Topics
- Practical session putting theory into practice
- Structuring the interview
- Developing questions
- Role play
- Constructive feedback

Suggested Method of Delivery
In-house programme delivered using organisational policy and procedure and advertised through the training prospectus.

Suggested Competence Measures
Question and answer.
Role play.

Recruitment and selection: M007B

Rationale
To develop the knowledge and skills of managers, supervisors and team leaders about the need for a systematic process for recruitment and selection, reducing the pitfalls and poor practice that could result in a financial implication for the organisation.

Employment legislation and ACAS codes of practice reinforce the need to train managers in the use of fair procedures for recruiting new staff and to prevent discrimination in selection procedures. It is also a requirement in line with organisational policy.

Staff Group
All staff who have responsibility for recruitment and selection in their work area, in particular all newly appointed staff with responsibility for recruitment and selection.

Frequency
As and when the policy is updated and/or amended.

Topics
- The recruitment and selection process
- Job descriptions and person specifications
- Preparing for interview
- Questioning techniques
- Interviewing skills

Suggested Method of Delivery
In-house programme delivered using organisational policy and procedure and advertised through the training prospectus.

Suggested Competence Measures
Question and answer.
Role play.

Personal development review (appraiser): M008A

Rationale
To develop the knowledge and skills of all staff managers, supervisors and team leaders about good practice, the purpose, benefits and process of appraisal and personal development planning.

Organisational policy requires all employees to have an annual review.

NB: for NHS organisations only – IWL, CHI standards and HR in the NHS Plan all emphasise the importance of all employees participating in the personal development review/ appraisal process.

Staff Group
All those with responsibility for carrying out appraisal reviews. Newly appointed managers, supervisors and team leaders.

Frequency
On commencement and as and when the policy is updated and/or amended.

Topics
- Context, purpose, benefits and process of appraisal
- Documentation
- Skills, knowledge and approach
- Setting objectives
- Giving performance feedback
- Personal development planning
- Managing the review meeting

Suggested Method of Delivery
In-house programme delivered using organisational policy and procedure and advertised through the training prospectus.

Suggested Competence Measures
Question and answer.
Role play.

Personal development review (appraisees): M008B

Rationale
To develop the knowledge and skills of all staff about good practice, the purpose, benefits and process of appraisal and personal development planning.

Organisational policy requires all employees to have an annual review.

NB: for NHS organisations only – IWL, CHI standards and HR in the NHS Plan all emphasise the importance of all employees participating in the personal development review/appraisal process.

Staff Group
All those who will undergo appraisal/performance review.

Frequency
On commencement and as and when the policy is updated and/or amended.

Topics
- Context, purpose, benefits and process of appraisal
- Documentation
- Skills, knowledge and approach
- Setting objectives
- Receiving performance feedback
- Personal development planning
- The review meeting

Suggested Method of Delivery
In-house programme delivered using organisational policy and procedure and advertised through the training prospectus.

Suggested Competence Measures
Question and answer.
Role play.

Clinical risk, adverse events, informing patients: M009

Rationale
Clinical negligence standards state that all employees with responsibility in these areas should be trained appropriately.

Staff Group
All qualified clinical staff who are involved in assessing and managing clinical risk, clinical adverse events, information to patients about interventions and treatments and obtaining consent, e.g. medical and nursing staff, occupational therapists, certain speech and language therapists, dieticians, dentists, psychologists, carers, counsellors.

Frequency
This will vary according to need and risk assessment but should be completed within three months of commencement in post with an update/refresher following any major changes to requirements.

Topics
- Clinical risk assessment and management and related policy and procedures, e.g. discharge planning
- The protection of the public and service users versus positive risk taking
- Assessment of patients for the possibility of self-harm or harm to others
- Managing the risk of self-harm or harm to others by service users
- Accessing and giving information about interventions to patients, including the risks and benefits
- Capability, consent and specific procedures, e.g. medicines

- Clinical adverse events, e.g. drug errors
- Disseminating and learning the lessons and acting on these
- Informing patients when an adverse event occurs that involves them
- Informing carers and/or relatives when an adverse event occurs involving their loved one

Suggested Method of Delivery
Courses advertised through training prospectus.

Suggested Competence Measures
Question and answer.
Scenarios.

Handling violence and aggression: M010 (generic)

Rationale
To ensure that all staff working with the public are aware of the procedures and advice given on handling violence and aggression in the workplace.

Staff Group
All staff.

Frequency
One off.

Topics
- Understanding fear and anger
- Assessing risks
- Personal safety/protecting yourself
- Managing confrontation and unpredictability
- Working alone
- Visiting homes
- Surviving outbursts

Suggested Methods of Delivery
In-house session by specialist.
External training programme.

Suggested Competence Measures
Scenarios.
Role play.
Oral test.

Handling violence and aggression: M010A (nursing specific)

Rationale
Current guidelines underpinning standards for training:
    Royal College of Nursing Institute
    Health Circular 76.11
    Nursing and Midwifery Council

The standards recommend varying levels of training targeted at different staff groups according to need.

Staff Group
Level 1 – all staff who may come into contact with members of the public and patients.
Level 2 – staff involved in lone working situations or working in clinical areas and therefore exposed to the general public and/or patients more frequently, e.g. working with older adults, learning disabilities, mental health and forensics.

Frequency
On commencement and every year thereafter (annual update and refresher).

Topics
Varying levels of training targeted at different staff groups according to needs.
● *Level 1* – personal safety/customer care
● *Level 2* – breakaway training/personal safety/lone working

Cont.

Suggested Method of Delivery
Programmes at all levels are tailored to meet the specific needs of directorates/specialties by arrangement.

Suggested Competence Measures
Simulation.
Role play.
Questionnaires.

Budgetary control: M011

Rationale
This session ensures that anyone with budgetary control/ responsibilities is aware of the processes and procedures involved in sound resource management.

Staff Group
Anyone with budgetary responsibilities.

Frequency
One off.

Topics
- Financial structures and governance
- Budgetary control
- Zero-based budgeting
- Creating efficiency savings

Suggested Methods of Delivery
In-house session by specialist.
External training provider.

Suggested Competence Measures
Question and answer.
In-tray exercise.

Client-focused service: M012

Rationale
To ensure that the workforce understands the priority given to internal and external clients (customers) and how services are geared to meet their needs.

Staff Group
Whole workforce.

Frequency
One off.

Topics
- Understanding the concept of client-focused service
- Identifying internal and external clients
- The importance of consistency
- Clear and concise communication
- User involvement and consultation

Suggested Methods of Delivery
In-house session by specialist.
External training programme.

Suggested Competence Measures
Question and answer.
Role play.

Supervisory training: M013

Rationale
The programme provides the basic skills and knowledge required by first-time supervisors to supervise the work of others effectively and in line with organisational policy.

Staff Group
First-time supervisors and team leaders.

Frequency
One off.

Topics
- The role of the supervisor
- Key responsibilities and limits of authority
- Establishing respect and trust in the team
- Identification of problems and solutions
- Understanding the policies and procedures related to managing a team
- Planning and scheduling work
- Prioritising work
- Applying planning techniques to formalise service delivery

Suggested Methods of Delivery
Internal programme.
External (generic) programme.

Suggested Competence Measure
Accredited test.

Management training: M014

Rationale
To ensure that management within the organisation is consistent and of a high standard, all managers will undertake this core skills management development programme.

Staff Group
All new managers and managers new to the organisation who do not hold a basic management qualification.

Frequency
One off.

Topics
- Roles and responsibilities of a manager
- Decision making and problem solving
- Project management methodology
- Setting objectives
- People management skills
- Communication skills
- Information management
- Resource management

Suggested Methods of Delivery
Internal programme.
External (generic) programme.

Suggested Competence Measure
Accredited test.

Audit and evaluation: M015

Rationale
In order for the organisation to operate effectively, it is vital to promote good, evidence-based practice and strive for continuous improvement. This can only be achieved if the organisation has robust audit and evaluation protocols that are actioned by the workforce.

Staff Group
Anyone involved in audit, evaluation of service or service reviews.

Frequency
One off.

Topics
- The audit cycle
- Gathering data
- Data sources
- Validity
- Interpreting data
- Analysis and presenting information

Suggested Methods of Delivery
In-house session.
External programme.

Suggested Competence Measures
Simulation.
In-tray exercise.
Action learning.

Appendices

Appendix 1: Local induction checklist

Have you covered the following on the day of commencement?	Completed ✓ or n/a
Introduction to work colleagues, mentor, clinical supervisor, etc.	
Availability of information about the organisation — annual report, business plan, staff handbook, etc.	
Confirmation of hours of work, shifts, rotas, etc.	
Confirmation of method of pay, pay and query point	
Complete commencement form, obtaining from employee: • birth certificate and NI number and/or P45 • evidence of qualification/professional registration documents/marriage certificate	
Checked the validity of the registration documents	
Explanation of uniform requirements and facilities	
Issue of keys and security arrangements for use of them	
Location of facilities, e.g. toilets, locker and eating	
Location of personnel policy file and how it can be accessed	
Location of clinical procedures file	
Car parking facilities	

Have you covered the following on the day of commencement?	Completed ✓ or n/a
Accident reporting procedure	
Departmental risks and health & safety responsibilities	
Fire evacuation procedure	
Name badge. ID badge issued	
Issue of diary	
Confirmation of organisational induction arrangements	

Employee's signature .... Date ......

Manager's signature .... Date ......

Have you covered the following within one week of commencement?	Completed ✓ or n/a
Annual leave entitlements and arrangements	
Standards/codes of conduct and behaviour	
Timekeeping standards	
Confidentiality	
Personal hygiene standards	
How they obtain personal employment number	
Educational facilities and opportunities	
First aid provision, boxes, personnel	
Occupational health facility	
Sickness reporting procedure	
Medical emergency procedure	
COSHH regulations	
Security arrangements	
Complaints procedure	
Team briefing	
FIP/mileage returns	
Lease car	
Standing financial instructions/fraud	
Staff carers network	
Staff benefits/discounts	
Disciplinary policy	

Have you covered the following within one week of commencement?	Completed ✓ or n/a
Grievance policy	
Safety policy	
Special leave	
Equal opportunities	
Trade union information	
Harassment	
Appraisal	

Employee's signature . . . . Date . . . . . .

Manager's signature . . . . Date . . . . . .

Within two months of commencement	*Date completed*
A statement of particulars	
Training on:	
Patient manual handling	
Food hygiene	
Infection control	
Data protection	
Safety on VDUs	

Employee's signature . . . . Date . . . . . .

Manager's signature . . . . Date . . . . . .

NB: TO BE RETAINED ON EMPLOYEE FILE.

Appendix 2: New employees and annual appraisal checklist

Name . . . . Department . . . .

Directorate . . . .

Employee number . . . . Review date. . . . .

This checklist should be used at PDR/appraisal by the manager and employee to identify annual training requirements for mandatory training. The checklist should be completed in conjunction with the relevant organisation guidelines, which will help determine relevant mandatory training for each member of staff depending on job role and responsibilities.

Shaded boxes denote that training is statutory for all staff.

The appraisal discussion should identify whether there is a need for refresher or update training in each subject area.

Topic	Date last undertaken	Update needed?
General health & safety induction training (including COSHH & RIDDOR)		
Departmental/role-specific health & safety instruction		
Fire safety		
Workplace risk assessment		
Manual handling: Back awareness Patients		
Infection control and sharps		
Cardiopulmonary resuscitation/ anaphylaxis		
First aid		
Food hygiene		
Confidentiality, Caldicott and complaints		
Data security and confidentiality		
Equality and diversity		
Whistleblowing and fraud		
Child protection		
Major incident planning		
Electrical testing		
VDU assessment		
Waste management		
General organisational induction		

Topic	Date last undertaken	Update needed?
Departmental induction		
Handling discipline at work		
Grievances and disputes		
Managing attendance		
Harassment and bullying		
Recruitment interviewing skills		
Recruitment and selection procedures		
Personal development review: Appraiser Appraisee		
Clinical risk, adverse events		
Handling violence and aggression: Generic Nursing specific		
Budgetary control		
Client-focused service		
Supervisory training		
Management training		
Personal development review/appraisal		

Date . . . .

Employee's signature: . . . .

Manager's signature: . . . .

Copies should also be retained for the employee's personal file and personal development portfolio.

Appendix 3: Sample training matrices

Sample matrix – mandatory training

Mandatory training	Whole workforce	Support staff	Team leaders	Managers	Professional staff
Induction, organisation M001	✓				
Induction, departmental M002	✓				
Handling discipline M003			✓	✓	
Grievance and disputes M004			✓	✓	
Managing attendance M005			✓	✓	
Harassment and bullying M006			✓	✓	
Recruitment interviewing M007A			✓	✓	✓

Mandatory training	Whole workforce	Support staff	Team leaders	Managers	Professional staff
Recruitment and selection M007B			✓	✓	✓
Appraiser M008A		✓ If appropriate	✓	✓	✓
Appraisee M008B	✓				
Clinical risk/adverse events M009			✓	✓	✓
Handling violence and aggression M010	✓				✓
Budgetary control M011				✓	
Client-focused service M012	✓	✓	✓		✓
Supervisory training M013			✓		✓ If appropriate
Management training M014				✓	✓ If appropriate
Audit and evaluation M015		✓	✓	✓	✓

Sample matrix – statutory training

Statutory training	Whole workforce	Support staff	Team leaders	Managers	Professional staff
H&S induction S001	✓				
H&S induction S002		✓	✓		
COSHH S003	✓				
RIDDOR S004	✓				
Fire safety S005	✓				
Workplace risk assessment S006				✓	✓
Manual handling: back awareness S007A		✓		✓	
Manual handling: patients S007B			✓		✓
Infection control S008	✓				
CPR/anaphylaxis S009	✓				
First aid S010		✓ Nominated			
Confidentiality S012	✓				

Statutory training	Whole workforce	Support staff	Team leaders	Managers	Professional staff
Data security S013		✓		✓	✓
Equity and diversity S014	✓				
Whistleblowing and fraud S015	✓				
Child protection: level 1 S016	✓				
Child protection: level 2 S017			✓	✓	✓
Child protection: level 3 S018			✓	✓	✓
Major incident planning S019			✓	✓	✓
Electrical testing O20		✓ Nominated			
VDU assessment S021		✓ Nominated			
Waste management S022		✓ Nominated			

Appendix 4: Statutory and mandatory training checklist

Statutory/mandatory unit	✓ or ×	Provider known	Gap
New starters General induction			
Departmental induction			
General health & safety induction			
Departmental/role-specific health & safety instruction			
COSHH			
RIDDOR			
Fundamental skills First aid			
Fire safety sessions/updates			
Workplace risk assessment			
Manual handling: back awareness			
Manual handling: patients			
Infection control/sharps			

Statutory/mandatory unit	✓ or ✗	Provider known	Gap
CPR/anaphylaxis			
Client-focused service			
Role-specific skills Food hygiene			
Data security and confidentiality			
Confidentiality, Caldicott Regulations and complaints			
Handling violence and aggression			
Clinical risk, adverse events, informing patients			
Budgetary control			
Electrical testing			
VDU assessment			
Waste management			
Audit and evaluation			
Managing people Handling discipline at work			
Grievance and disputes			
Supervisory training Management training			
Managing attendance			
Recruitment and selection			
Recruitment interviewing skills			

Statutory/mandatory unit	✓ or ✗	Provider known	Gap
Personal development review/appraisal: Appraiser Appraisee			
Policies and legislation Equality and diversity			
Harassment and bullying			
Whistleblowing and fraud			
Child protection			
Major incident planning			
IT training			
European Computer Driving Licence (ECDL)			

Appendix 5: Significant event analysis template

	Detail	Result
Event to be analysed		

Issues	Actions	Result
How was the event managed initially?		
Who was involved?		
What were the positive things that occurred?		
What were the negative things that occurred?		
Could anyone else have contributed positively to the event?		
How could they?		
What were the key factors that determined this outcome?		
Were there any interface issues?		
Were there any team issues?		
Follow-up arrangements		

What action/policy decision will you take as a result of this analysis?

Who will be responsible for ensuring this is done?

When will the task be completed?

Appendix 6:
Risk assessment form

Risk being assessed	
Likelihood of risk occurring	
Who is involved?	
Preventative steps taken	
Options to reduce/eliminate risk	
Action taken	
Date – signed	Next review date

Appendix 7:
Generic statutory and
mandatory training
policy (sample)

1   Policy statement

[The organisation] is committed to creating a learning organisation where its staff are recognised as its most important resource and their learning is valued, supported and shared, to enable continuous quality improvement and the highest standards of safe and effective patient care delivered consistently.

This policy applies to all staff, full and part-time staff, job sharers, those on temporary and fixed-term contracts, without discrimination.

[The organisation] will establish key systems and processes that support safe and competent practice throughout the organisation and across all professions and staff groups.

Empirical learning

- An organisation-wide staff performance and development scheme that requires all staff members to undertake an annual appraisal, track their statutory and mandatory training status and produce a personal development plan highlighting their development needs and planned activity to meet those needs.

- Those needs are matched with corporate performance objectives and service delivery priorities and form the curriculum for training and education provision.

Ethical learning

- Through clinical governance, to operate a risk management process that feeds learning into the corporate planning cycle to ensure clinical effectiveness.
- To actively involve patients, users and carers in the development and shaping of services and to incorporate the learning into staff training and education programmes.
- To enhance ethical learning through such initiatives as the Patient Advice and Liaison Service (PALS), staff opinion surveys and the Expert Patient Programme (EPP).

Partnership learning

- Continue to develop links with other PCTs, local authorities, social services and the voluntary sector to contribute to and benefit from cross-boundary learning, education and training opportunities.
- To access multidisciplinary, cross-organisation training modules and programmes, in common areas such as statutory training, with other healthcare providers.
- To work with educational institutions and providers to develop curriculum and course content that meets the changing requirements of NHS organisations.

Core values of education, training and development

- To offer equitable and fair access to education, training and learning to the whole workforce.

- To support individuals and teams who use their learning as a means of continuous improvement and enable them to deliver the highest standards of patient care.
- Through the e-learning strategy, provide up-to-date, flexible resources and technology that support the education and training requirements of our workforce.
- To ensure that the focus for statutory and mandatory training is measuring competence of the individual to operate safely and competently, in accordance with trust policies and procedures.

2 Statutory and mandatory training standards

A set of standards has been agreed which details the direction of statutory and mandatory training for the organisation.

- All new staff to undertake a systematic induction programme during the first six months of their employment.
- Minimum statutory and mandatory training requirements assigned to each role/post holder in the organisation (for all staff groups) to include mandatory training, clinical updates, health & safety training, supervisory/management baseline training, professional development and personal development activities.
- Everyone to undertake an annual appraisal and identify training and development needs in a personal development plan.
- Minimum competency standards for generic areas, i.e. computer skills.
- All training and development activity to be measured by the participant using the organisation's evaluation process.

A mechanism for defining expectations

All supported learning to be defined through a learning contract establishing the learning objectives and outcomes of the participant and the support that will be provided by the organisation.

A process for systematic reflection

A process that captures identified development needs and learning outcomes and feeds them into the corporate planning activities of commissioning, service design, clinical effectiveness and delivery of care.

3   Definitions

For the purposes of this policy the following definitions apply.

The organisation is required by law to ensure that staff undertake training specific to the nature of their working environment (statutory training), e.g. health & safety training, fire lectures, etc. In addition, the organisation has published a list of its standard requirements for training (mandatory training) which all members of staff are subject to.

Statutory and mandatory training is about enabling staff to acquire the skills and knowledge to meet:

- statutory/mandatory and professional requirements (e.g. health & safety, CPD, etc.)
- the needs arising from their job description and personal objectives
- the needs arising from the changing role and priorities of the PCT (corporate objectives).

4   Responsibilities

- The organisation is responsible for providing opportunities for its workforce to meet their statutory and mandatory training and development needs, identified through the annual appraisal process within the available resources.

- Team co-ordinators and line managers are responsible for supporting individuals to identify their statutory and mandatory training needs during the annual appraisal process and helping to source the appropriate learning activity to meet those needs.
- Employees have a joint responsibility with their team co-ordinator/line manager to identify their statutory and mandatory training requirements. They are also required to undertake any training agreed as part of a corporate organisational development programme. Employees are also responsible for keeping their continuing professional development (CPD) portfolios up to date with certificates, awards and evaluation sheets that demonstrate continuing learning.
- Statutory and mandatory training is a critical component of everyone's role and failure to comply with minimum standards will be considered a breech of terms and conditions.

5 Allocation of resources

The organisation will endeavour to provide the necessary resources, i.e. budgets, staffing and management time, to enable employee development to be carried out in a timely and effective manner.

The allocation of resources for training and development will be determined by the organisation and will be based on the training plan, learning strategy and the organisation's priorities.

6 Annual appraisal interview

The organisation is committed to the continuing development of its valued workforce and a demonstration of that is the undertaking to give every member of staff the opportunity to undergo an annual appraisal meeting. This is a formative, developmental process that offers a review of the previous year's performance.

It provides each employee with the opportunity to understand corporate objectives for the coming year and formulate personal objectives in response. It also offers a systematic monitoring of statutory and mandatory training status and identification of training and development needs of the individual, to skill them to the appropriate level, enabling them to achieve agreed objectives.

As a result, training and development are targeted directly at need, making it an efficient and cost-effective process for the individual as well as the organisation.

7   Process

Every team co-ordinator/line manager has responsibility for conducting an annual appraisal meeting with each member of their staff (directly accountable to them). At the meeting a personal development plan (PDP) will be drawn up and agreed between the staff member and line manager. The PDP should identify:

- status of statutory and mandatory training
- training and development needs arising from the corporate objectives and PCT priorities
- training and development needs arising from the role, responsibilities, personal objectives and job description of the staff member
- training and development needs arising from personal development of career plans
- the objectives of training and development
- the training activity/method of training
- training activity source
- target date for achievement
- method of evaluation.

Ideally, a progress review should take place after six months to ensure the plan is still relevant and on target for achievement.

Where a member of staff changes their job or is promoted, their new team co-ordinator/line manager should undertake an appraisal to identify any training and development required to allow the person to undertake their new role and responsibilities. This training may take the form of coaching/structured handover by the team leader/line manager or the incumbent post holder. It may also require the member of staff to undertake external or professional training where necessary.

8 Corporate training

Where there is a need for training to meet a legal requirement (e.g. health & safety) or a corporate requirement (e.g. software training) or it is more cost effective to offer an in-house training programme (e.g. appraisal training), corporate training will be offered.

Induction training

To demonstrate to new employees how the organisation values its workforce and the contribution they make as an individual (not just as a post holder), a structured induction programme will be undertaken by all new employees to help them gain a feel for the philosophy of the organisation and to understand its values, beliefs and ethos. The induction will also help new members of staff to understand their role and responsibilities from day 1, easing them into the organisation. To help them through the early stages of their employment, each new staff member will be presented with an induction manual, tailored to their requirements and identified needs.

The organisation views the induction process as a fundamental tool in establishing a strong psychological contract with new employees. Induction is mandatory and a requirement of employment. The organisation considers induction best practice and a key factor in improving recruitment and retention practice.

Health & safety training

The organisation has certain responsibilities under statutory health & safety law to provide information, training, instruction and supervision to staff to ensure a safe working environment.

Mandatory and statutory training

Tables of statutory and mandatory training detail the requirements for different staff groups and post holders.

Supervisory and management training

All team leaders and managers will be offered the necessary training to enable them to supervise/manage their staff and related functions effectively. This includes the ability to conduct appraisals with their staff and the implementation of the organisation's induction process.

9   Monitoring of statutory and mandatory training

Prior to undertaking any training or development, an employee will have a short meeting with their team co-ordinator/line manager to identify the aims and objectives of the training. The relevant training approval form must be completed by both parties, recording the individual's needs and objectives and how these support their annual objectives and PDP. This is the learning contract.

After the training has taken place, a second short meeting (post-course review) should take place to discuss the transfer of new knowledge or skill into the workplace. At this time any additional support required to do this effectively should be agreed.

Individual staff members should include records of these meetings and copies of the learning contract in their CPD portfolio.

All training approval forms will be collated by the training co-ordinator to ensure that the organisation has an accurate picture of training activity and can operate budgetary management controls. An annual report will be issued detailing training undertaken, organisational benefits, costs and future investment plans.

Evaluation process

Monitoring the effectiveness of training and development activities is a critical element and a process is outlined in the organisation's education and training policy.

Travel and accommodation

Expenses should be kept to a minimum wherever possible and persons attending the same programme (where possible) should travel together. The driver may then apply for 100% reimbursement at public transport rate for mileage above their normal workbase mileage.

Staff required to travel by train can apply for a travel card warrant or purchase standard-class rail tickets.

All travel claims should be completed using a standard travel expenses form.

Staff requiring overnight accommodation in a hotel/guest house, with the agreement of their line manager, will be reimbursed as follows:

- bed and breakfast up to a normal limited rate of £55 per night
- a meals allowance of £20 to cover the cost of a main evening meal and one other day-time meal
- staff who are on authority business after 7.30pm are allowed £15 subsistence allowance for an evening meal.

Study leave

It is important for all staff to have access to the training and development they need and that the organisation offers support to them whilst they study. To ensure fair access for education and training, there are guidelines that establish levels of reimbursement and how to apply for training and development.

Training programmes include short courses, clinical updates, mandatory training, conferences, etc.

Gaining approval for study leave/training

This is described simply in the flow chart below.

Individual staff member to identify training need

↓

Discuss with your locality/line manager (link to PDP)

↓

Provisionally book a place on course

↓

Complete study leave form

↓

Send to locality/line manager

↓

Below £500 total cost: locality manager to authorise payment from locality/line manager budget

↓

Above £500 total cost: locality manager to send study leave form to relevant director for authorisation (attach copy of PDP)

↓

Director to make decision regarding authorisation for funding and inform locality/line manager

↓

Confirmation of approval to be sent to individual by training co-ordinator (copy to locality/line manager)

(Process needs reviewing and re-publicising throughout the organisation.)

Index

Page numbers in *italics* refer to illustrations or tables.
Page numbers in **bold** refer to checklists and proformas (Appendices).